A THYROID AND HORMONE DIET

BY

Susan Seymour

First published March 2001

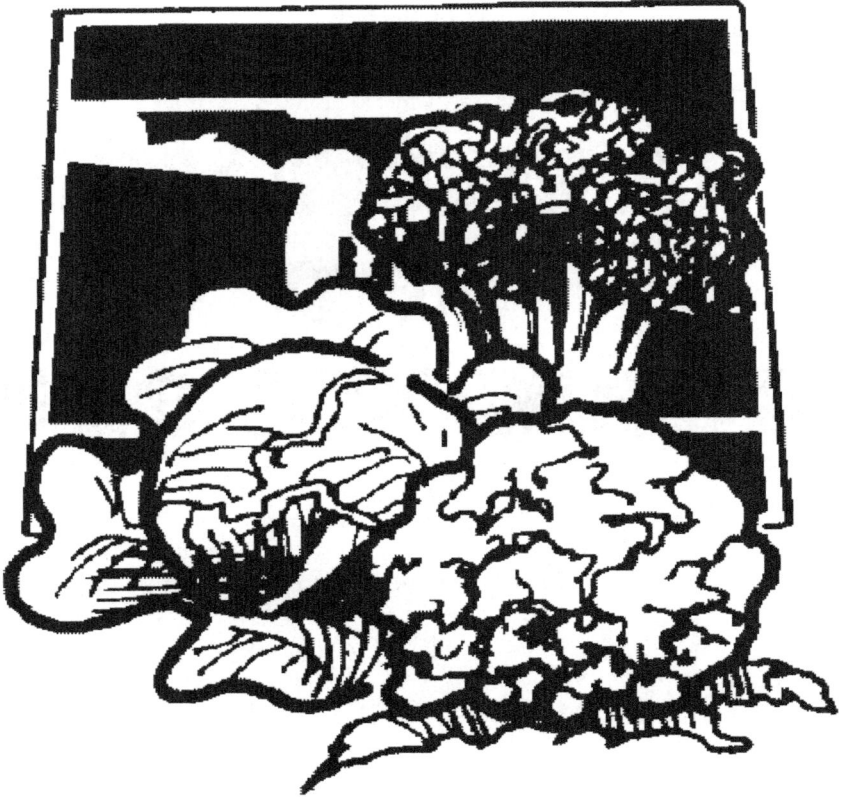

"Yummy lovely cabbages?" Are they the right food for thyroid wellness?

Read how to get back to nature and heal yourself. Contains advice on recipes, food suggestions, chemicals, and poisons in everyday foods that make us ill, how they affect the thyroid and make us sick. Examples: "Do you know lipstick contains barium?", "Do you know fluoride is more poisonous than lead and only slightly less toxic to arsenic?"

CONTENTS

CHAPTER ONE – THE BEGINNING

"Eat your greens; they are good for you" I hear in my head and on television.

Ever wondered why children do not like greens in general? They know instinctively that they are NOT good for you – just the opposite. If you have low thyroid function they can make matters very much worse. Remember the gassy tummy from those sprouts? Wondered why it happened? The answer lies in the composition of the cabbage family. They include cabbage, spring greens, radish, mustard, cauliflower, sprouts, broccoli etc. The brassica family contain chemicals called progoitrins – which means literally makes goitres.

Most plants contain hormones and chemicals or they begin a hormonal reaction. If eaten wisely they can enhance your well-being 100%. If abused; either intentionally or unintentionally our guts can become exhausted, full of bacteria, moulds, fungus, candida, and parasites. The older we are the more our gut needs attention. If we are wise then sayings like "bowel cleanse" "detox" and "digestive enzymes" will become part of our lives.

Why do we need a bowel cleanse? Answer; is to get rid of old parasites and their discharge, to clean out old foods clinging to the walls of our bowels, and to heal us. How often do we need to do this? The answer is once or twice a year.

Why do we need to detox? The answer is to cleanse our food processing system and start afresh. Also to get rid of those unwanted guests and food poisoning bacteria moulds and fungus in our gut.

What are digestive enzymes? Answer; they help us break down our foods and absorb the nutrients easily.

These simple procedures should be undertaken before any diet begins.

So why is the thyroid diet different from others you may ask? Certain foods affect different aspects of our lives. Carbohydrates boost energy for a short time, but exhausts adrenal glands in the long run. Wheat and grains pass through in our gut in 20 minutes – this is not long enough to feed us until the next meal time. It is this process that makes us constantly hungry. Carbohydrates, starches, and sugars create hyper-insulinism; which is an excess of insulin. Insulin can lay down as fat and reduces adrenal function. (Adrenals glands are two hat-like glands that sit atop of our kidneys making steroid hormones and keeping us alive). Remember our cells are mostly protein and fat and protein heals.

Many of those who become hypothyroid do so because of incorrect diet which drains the adrenals, reducing their function and then the thyroid declines too. That is why blood tests for thyroid often do not show the illness in its' true light. The thyroid needs the steroid hormones to make it work. Constant stress leaves the cortisol and DHEA hormones too low, the patient becomes exhausted, and so does the thyroid. This is called secondary hypothyroidism, and no amount of blood tests for thyroid will show this clearly. By the time the patient is below "borderline" they are critical and have a poor quality of life.

The objective of this book is to link the hormones to the food we eat, and to show how this downward spiral can stop if you want it to.

The key to the thyroid diet is that everyone is different and everyone cannot eat the same foods. Some people are extremely toxic to wheat, as are many blood group O people. It can give you palpitations, feelings of hot then too cool. It can also interfere with sleeping patterns, and is generally a pain to live with because virtually everything has wheat added. Corn is not much better and rye, (which I used as an alternative) is often a nightmare. Our western diet is awash with wheat, and when you consider almost 50% of the population is blood group O, we are in trouble. Wheat can put on a pound overnight. Some doctors laugh at this and say it is impossible. You need to think of what wheat does in water, (swells) it is not surprising that we swell too.

It is common for people to refuse to give up wheat, and it has to be accepted that they are resigned to being ill. That is something hard to understand.

On a personal note:

I also know more who have given it up and lost inches and pounds. A lady from Blackpool came to see me she showed up as having a biological age of 80, but was just aged 62. Her legs felt heavy she was tired; at one point she could not walk down the road without holding on to a wall. People thought she was drunk because she frequently fell over. She had spent years of going to the doctor and he had spent years of going to see her, because she was so ill she could not get off the sofa. So what happened? She changed her diet and her lifestyle, and within six weeks her biological age dropped to 30! Her body shrunk. She looked ten, if not more, years younger. The light came back into her life. Her weight fell off; she was overjoyed and so was I. I consider her a ray of light in a sometimes dark world of disbelief. Her belief in me is something I both cherish and thank her for. Then there are the others – impatient because it does not happen quickly enough. They do not persevere are weak willed and loose sight of their goal; which is to get well and lead something of a normal life again.

THE BOWEL CLEANSE

So where do we begin? Firstly buy some psyllium hulls/husks, (HEALTHY BOWELS) from the health food shop. Take half a teaspoon in mineral water at night before you go to bed. The texture is different but they are neutral, and the body usually welcomes them energetically. They go through the gut, intestines, and bowel gently scraping away the old food clinging to the walls. Parasites and their discharges are also swept out. Bacteria and moulds may need the detox too but the hulls do a good job of cleaning the system. It is not unusual to have the runs at some points after a day or so. Do not be worried by this as it is your system cleaning all the rubbish out from it. The large intestine time is between four and six during the night – so don't be surprised if it happens then. Morning is the most usual.

Drink plenty of mineral water and lemon juice while this is happening. You do feel as though your insides are falling out so try to do this over a four day period when life is not busy. If you cannot stand the texture of the hulls they do come in capsule form, and are as good, if a little more expensive.

Alternatives to the neat psyllium hulls are – hulls in capsule form
A medium detox or paracleanse is made up of mild herbs.

The Chinese detox uses stronger herbs in capsule form – you take six at night for three to seven days.

A thorough detox would be a 14 night paracleanse, repeated in 2 weeks to kill the eggs. Always start on the full moon when they are at their most active. Have two weeks off and repeat.

The experts say we absorb around a kilo of parasites per year, either by breathing them in or eating them.

THE DETOX

I do not advocate starvation for anyone. It usually causes reverse T3, (which is the energy hormone). That is not what any detox means. Take two sticks of celery, a small handful of blue berries and half a lemon. Add to this some off the boil Evian water and a quarter teaspoon of bicarbonate of soda. Liquidise well and strain. Dilute half and half with Evian, and drink a small glass every two hours for four days or longer.

In addition to this eat fresh organic fruit and vegetables with a small quantity of protein. Use a juicer if you prefer – but do not have more than five glasses of juiced fruit and vegetables per day. Do not mix fruit and vegetables. Eat or drink separately. Eat absolutely NO processed food or dairy. That means is man made it avoid it. Do not take any supplements; vitamins or minerals during this time. Remember it is only for four days but you can do it regularly if it helps.

DIGESTIVE ENZYMES

Why do we need them? The simple answer is that as we get older we have less and less of them. They are vital to break down our food so that it can be absorbed properly. Remember all those red hot cups of tea? They are so destructive to the pancreatic and digestive enzymes; burning them away. The Chinese say that food should be warm – not hot and not cold. They also say you should not eat cold food in winter and vice versa. Some foods are hot even when they are cold – like chillies. Some foods are cold even when they are hot like peppermint tea. We are either yin or yang people in our make up and our body parts are also yin and yang. Yin is the soft parts like our organs. Yang is the hard parts like our bones. Food compatibility varies because of this.

When you have done the detox, bowel cleanse, and started the digestive enzymes choosing your food is next.

The basis of any diet is how to shop. First do not shop when you are hungry. This is for two reasons. One your food bill will be higher, and two you will add things to your basket/trolley that should not be there. Do your shopping half to 2 hours after eating. Where to shop is the next question. There are farmers markets in most parts of the country. Here you can buy cheap organic produce. Or look in yellow pages. Why organic? Pesticides are very unhealthy for us. Fruits in particular are sprayed with pesticides some like grapes up to six times in their life on the vine. In order to have the purest diet organic is the way forward.

What should we buy? The third rule is the best - in equal parts - protein, fruits, and vegetables. Plus those foods you are NOT toxic or have an allergy to. As the body heals it becomes stronger and can tolerate more food types.

Water is the biggest problem. DO NOT DRINK TAP WATER. Why? It contains chloride, which is carcinogenic and sometimes cryptosporidium, (a parasite from sheep washed down in the water table from their faeces and urine), but most deadly is the fluoride. Fluoride is more toxic than lead and only marginally less toxic than arsenic. In other words do not put it in your mouth. Unfortunately you will have to wash in it. If I am visiting a poor water area I always rinse my mouth and face in mineral water. Fluoride interferes with thyroid function – remember the gagging after cleaning your teeth? Canada is the worlds leading country for research into fluoride poisoning. For more details contact the Pure Water Association in Yorkshire. Canada has some good websites for research into toxic water.

So which mineral water to choose? Volvic is best. Read the labels – if it has high nitrates reject it, same with fluoride (yes some brands do put it in). Perrier has its' own unique energy level.

Learn how to read labels. Tesco have a new range of organic products – however their wheat products contain preservative so avoid – even without the wheat.

The no list should contain: sweets, mints, tea, coffee, sugar, flour, bread, wheat, pasta, margarine, etc.

Have a budget and stick to it. Write out your list of foods that you have been tested for that balance you, and keep it in your purse, handbag, or wallet. If it is on the yes list then that is what you have tested positive to balance you. Avoid all others for now.

"LIFE'S A BREEZE"

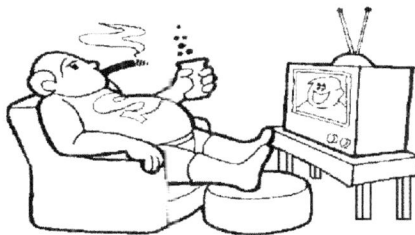

(UNTIL THE HEART ATTACK)

CHAPTER TWO – FOODS

ADVERTISING BRAINWASHING

As you snuggle down for a comfy night in front of the television life seems so informed. "Eat wheat and have a healthy heart" the adverts tell us. Drink coke, smell lovely, have a clean home etc. We are told constantly to eat a high fibre diet, and keep fats low if not eradicated all together.

The cholesterolitis that is sweeping the country is bad for our health. Why? All hormones are made from cholesterol. Cutting out fat does not ultimately reduce cholesterol. (See Dr. Atkins Age-defying Diet). Cutting out carbohydrates should.

A high wheat, fibre, and carbohydrate diet will only do one thing – make you fat. In the short term you may loose weight but in the long term your hormones will be reduced and – sorry – that means more good fats and oils. Hormones keep your metabolism regulated, help your food to digest, and they keep you alive. Hormones also make you thin.

So where do we begin? And what do foods do?

Each person is an individual. Each tummy and gut is individual to that person. If we were all alike we would look like clones of each other, eat the same foods, and have the same tastes. But we are not. What one person likes does not suit another. Often we do not know why we hate some foods, as we get older our tolerance becomes even more stressed, and some foods are avoided because they upset us.

All people (and animals) should be food tested. Food is a medicine. I know it is to be enjoyed and some people live for that enjoyment, nevertheless food means FEED. On the downside food can also mean a type of poison to us.

Coke, (almost acid 2.5 pH), is currently one of the worlds' top selling brands. Coke contains aspartame, which stops the pituitary from working properly. (The pituitary makes TSH – thyroid stimulating hormone). The number of people who have tummy problems caused by drinking coke is amazing. It raises stomach acid to levels which are simply unacceptable.

Other foods contain aspartame – always check the labels on pre-prepared foods. Avoid ALL E- numbers, colours, preservative, and additives Eat organic – but check the labels as some organic foods contain preservatives.

You can dowse food with a pendulum to see if it suits you. A needle on cotton acts as a good pendulum. On a dowsing scale foods vary from 1 – 40. 40 being death. Rosemary and lavender are 3 and 4 respectively. Apple is a ten. Alcohol and aluminium are at 26. Tomato is 38 and potato is 39. The higher the number the more stressed the body becomes. Anything over 20 is usually putting the body out of balance.

Dowsing is a crude alternative to EAV (point testing). An alternative is to use Kinesiology. Hold your right arm out to the side. Get someone to hold food to your tummy and press down on your arm. If you cannot hold a resistance then that food may weaken you.

Some people are citrus toxic, although I know of only one who is toxic to lemons. The lemon is the best anti-oxidant we have. Look at what it does to fruits – they do not go brown (rusty) as a reaction to oxygen. Lemons have the same effect on you. Please buy organic or wax free, natural ones though, not something you squeeze out of a plastic lemon, this has preservative in it. An easy way to get the juice from a lemon is to roll it first on a hard surface until it becomes soft, and then make a little slit and squeeze hard. All the juice will run out easily into your glass. Lemons have the perfect pH (5)

Most shampoo and bath products have citric acid in them (so do fizzy drinks). If you are citrus toxic – perhaps blood group O – then avoid these. If it goes onto your skin then it goes into your body transdermally, (through the skin), so take care to have all these products tested too.

The elimination diet is not welcomed by most, yet after three days painkillers are consigned to the cupboard permanently, sleeping becomes more regular, gassy bloated tummy's go down, the runs subside and life begins to return to normal.

The basis of the thyroid diet is to eat small meals on a regular basis. This means keeping the metabolism up constantly. By avoiding sugars, carbohydrates, caffeine, and alcohol the blood sugar peaks and troughs begin to level out. Hypoglycaemia is the enemy of hypothyroids and by eliminating sugar etc. this distressing condition eases. Also candida lives on sugars and starches. Many hypothyroids have a problem with this. Chromium helps with low blood sugar.

The average person cannot or will not give up wheat. Many people are toxic to it, and cannot understand that it is the

. MOST ageing food one can eat. When wheat is put into our stomachs the adrenals have to work overtime to pump out hormones to stimulate digestion. The result is that the adrenals become exhausted. Add to this an allergy to wheat and the adrenals are pumping out high quantities of anti-histamines too. So if you wonder why you feel sleepy after eating carbohydrates this is one of the answers. The other is the release of brain hormones.

Look at what rice and grains do in water. They swell up. You are 70% water and don't think you are an exception - you will still swell up. Even the slim actress's say their tummies became flatter when she gave up wheat. Of course the glamorous stars also do not eat high carbohydrates, in interviews they eloquently say they (carbohydrates), are ageing and not to eat them. What is meant is not an excess of starchy foods like potatoes bread etc. Most foods contain some carbohydrate.

So the argument is that we need SOME carbs in our diet. Most foods like milk, carrots etc contain carbohydrates. See Dr. Atkins "The New Diet" book for details. The glycaemic index is on page 312. Peanuts have a 13 rating, glucose and maltose are the highest at 110. Grapefruit is 26 and orange is 40. Rice, bread etc are around the 70 mark.

What do we do first, where do we begin and how to shop for the right foods. We also need to understand that our loved ones probably do not need to go on the exclusion thyroid diet, as they are may feel well. They may however like to support you and be food tested to, and join you in your quest for wellness.

It takes some time for our digestive tracts to heal. Once parasites and bacteria are cleansed out the gut needs time to repair itself. Don't expect miracles in the first week, although some do happen.

By the end of the six week protocol you should be feeling like you can cope with life again, and if not something else needs to be done.

The next chapter is the Atkins Diet in brief. At each meal your plate should be one third protein, (the size of your palm), two thirds vegetables and 1oz good oil or butter.

In the Atkins New Diet Revolution book he says you can drink diet fizzy drinks. Do not do this as your body can be starved of oxygen without putting more carbon dioxide into it. Avoid all processed or industrial foods.

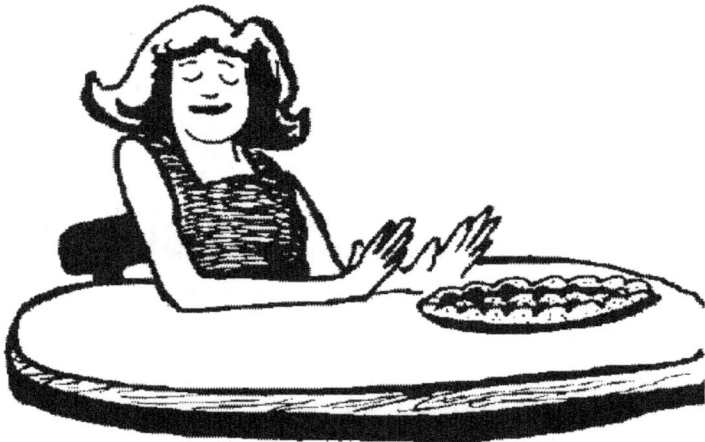

The Atkins Diet

CHAPTER THREE

What is The Atkins Diet?

It's a lifetime nutritional philosophy; focusing on the consumption of nutrient-dense, unprocessed foods and vita-nutrient supplementation. The Atkins diet restricts processed/refined carbohydrates (which make up over 50% of many people's diets), such as high-sugar foods, breads, pasta, cereal, and starchy vegetables. Core vita-nutrient supplementation includes a full-spectrum multi-vitamin and an essential oils/fatty acid formula.

Atkins tested the diet for over 30 years and it has been embraced by an estimated 20 million people worldwide since the release of Dr. Atkins' Diet Revolution in the 1970s. The cornerstone of the treatment protocols for over 60,000 patients of The Atkins Centre for Complementary Medicine in New York City.

The Major Benefits of the Diet:
Diets high in sugar and refined carbohydrates like bread, pasta, cereal, and other mainly 'low-fat' processed foods increase your body's production of insulin. When insulin is at high levels in the body, the food you eat can get readily converted into body fat, in the form of triglycerides (to top it off, high triglyceride levels in the body is one of the greatest risk factors for heart disease).

Even worse, high carbohydrate meals tend to leave you less satisfied than those that contain adequate fat levels; so you eat more and get hungrier sooner. If you find this hard to believe, think about how much pasta you can eat at lunch and then how hungry you are running to the vending machine for another 'carbo-fix' in the mid-afternoon. If the pasta you ate was really giving your body what it needed, you would stay full until dinner time. So the typical low-protein, low-fat meal leaves you eating more and hungry sooner. Corn fed pigs in America put on more weight than those fed on protein, (Broda Barnes).

So what should you do?

Get off the insulin generating roller coaster of the low-fat diet and start cutting down on your carbohydrate consumption, especially the worst offenders: sugar, white flour and other refined carbohydrate-based products.

What can you expect from this?

The answer is dieting results, more energy, and a feeling of wellness.

Three wonderful results:

1. You'll start to burn fat for energy:

Since carbohydrates are the body's primary energy source, you'll rarely use your secondary energy source, you own body fat, for energy unless you restrict carbohydrate consumption. This offers a lifetime of body fat burning, which is the goal of most people trying to lose weight.

2. You won't feel hungry in between meals:

  The biggest battle that most people have with weight loss is
the constant obsession with food (for example, if you've ever
thought about dinner when you're eating lunch). Again, much
of this is caused by blood sugar fluctuations that are
aggravated by carbohydrate consumption (especially the
refined kind). By cutting the carbs, you'll maintain a more
even blood sugar level throughout the day. No more false
hunger pains or mid-afternoon brain drains.

3. Your overall health will improve and you'll feel better:

  Many of the toxins you take into your body are stored in
your fat cells. By getting your body to burn stored fat, you
allow it to clean it out. Combined with the benefits of stable
blood sugar, the end result is that many common ailments you
have been experiencing could well be alleviated. Fatigue,
irritability, depression, headaches, and even many forms of
joint and muscular pain simply go away. Furthermore, you
should see a significant improvement in your blood profile,
(including cholesterol and blood pressure levels). All this leads
to better health and a feeling of well-being, something all of
us strive to bring into our lives.

Key Information about Sugar

  It contains no vitamins. No minerals. It is 100%
carbohydrate. So it must be metabolized immediately. The
stores of nutrients built up in your body are called out like
militia men, to 'charge' the sugar, and similar forms like
glucose and fructose, and turn it into ready energy, depleting

your body in the process. Sugar is an energy sucker: the Anti-Nutrient.

White flour is its second-cousin, almost as bad. When you partner the two together, flour and sugar, it spells disaster for anyone trying to maintain a healthy body, let alone someone who is fighting disease or trying to lose weight. If they are consumed on a regular basis, the body is in a constant state of nutritional deficiency. If you don't believe that sugar is an anti-nutrient, try having a rich dessert after dinner on a night you're feeling under the weather, you'll be sure to wake up the next morning feeling you have a full-blown illness.

What's frightening is that in recent years, the government, and other advisory groups like the American Medical Association and BMA, have encouraged the consumption of flour by unveiling a new food pyramid that is based on grains and recommends six to eleven servings a day. And no distinction is made between white processed flour, which is stripped of the nutrients, especially important trace minerals, and the much healthier whole grains, (unless you have a food allergy).

The result is that some Americans and Britons now think they're making healthy choices by loading up on cereals, pasta, crackers, and breads. We even have products like toasting tarts with 39 grams of carbohydrate, 20 of which are sugar, carrying the American Heart Association Seal of Approval.

It is a travesty that such foods are recommended to us.

So how do we protect ourselves and stay healthy?

One thing we can do is eat a healthy, balanced diet of low-carbohydrate foods. And when our foods fail us, as they often do after being picked, shipped, stripped, processed and packaged, we can protect ourselves with solid vita-nutrient support. It is critical that you include this extra 'insurance policy' to take you into the kind of healthy life we all want to lead.

Answering the Critics

While mainstream medicine and nutrition have, on the whole, criticized the Atkins Diet, the facts speak for themselves:
Dr. Atkins and his colleagues at The Atkins Centre for Complementary Medicine in New York have already treated over 60,000 patients using the Atkins Diet as a primary protocol. These patients experience all the beneficial effects detailed above, as well as improved blood pressure, lower cholesterol, and a lower or completely eradicated dependence on prescription drugs. While the mainstream critics continue to lament the consumption of fat as the root of America and Britain's weight problem, only carbohydrate consumption, (mostly refined) has increased in the past few decades, while fat consumption has declined (as the **'low-fat/high carb' diet has been promoted as the best nutritional option for <u>every living person</u>**).

During this time:

Obesity, which in the past had consistently applied to about 25% of the population, increased to 33% Heart disease now accounts for 50% of all deaths, up from 40% in the 1970s.

Britain and USA have the highest (and rising) levels of heart disease and cancer.

Cases of diabetes are growing in near epidemic proportions (in fact, children are now contracting adult-onset diabetes). Hypertension, chronic fatigue, and attention-deficit-disorder are now well recognized conditions.

All of these conditions are linked not by the amount of fat in ones diet, but by blood sugar disturbances and insulin disorders caused by excessive refined carbohydrate consumption.

The average person now consumes over 150 pounds of sugar a year, up from less then 10 pounds in the 19th century). While medical and nutritional journals are filled with studies documenting the body's requirement of essential fatty acids and essential amino acids (derived from protein), there is no such thing as an essential carbohydrate. Why then does the FDA recommend an average of 16 servings a day?

The Atkins Diet is not a no-carbohydrate diet. The diet focuses on very limited consumption of the types of carbohydrates that tend to spike blood sugar levels the most, including non-whole grain bread, pastas, refined sugar products, juices, and high sugar/starchy fruits and vegetables. Atkins Dieters learn to determine their personal sensitivity to carbohydrates, as a way to manage their weight and health for life.

Scientific References Related to a Low-Carbohydrate Eating Philosophy (such as the Atkins Diet):

ON CANCER:

'Saturated fat was not associated with the risk of breast cancer'& 'we found no positive association between intake of total fat and risk of invasive breast cancer'.
*Reference: Wolk, A. et al, Archives of Internal Medicine 1998; 158:41-45

'We found no evidence of a positive association between total dietary fat intake and the risk of breast cancer. There was no reduction in risk even among women whose energy intake from fat was less than 20 percent of total energy intake. In the context of the Western lifestyle, lowering the total intake of fat in midlife is unlikely to reduce the risk of breast cancer substantially.'
*Reference: Hunter D. et al, New England Journal of Medicine,; 1996 334:356-61

'The risk of breast cancer decreased with increasing total fat intake (trend p0.01) whereas the risk increase with increasing intake of available carbohydrates (trend p=0.002)'& 'The findings also suggest a possible risk, in southern European populations, of reliance on a diet largely based on starch.'
*Reference: Franceschi S. et al, Lancet 1996; 347: 1351-56

'Sugar consumption is positively associated with cancer in humans and test animals.* Tumours are know to b enormous sugar absorbers.'
*Sally Fallon, Nourishing Traditions 1995 Promotion Publishing
*Reference: Beasley, Joseph D, MD and Jerry J Swift, MA The Kellogg Report, 1989 The Institute of Health Policy and Practice, Annandale-on-Hudson, New York, 129.

'Johns Hopkins researchers have found evidence that some cancer cells are such incredible sugar junkies that they'll self-destruct when deprived of glucose, their biological sweet of choice'...'Scientists have long suspected that the cancer cell's heavy reliance on glucose, its main source of strength and vitality, also could be one of its great weaknesses, and Dang's new results are among the most direct proofs yet of the idea.'

* Johns Hopkins Medical Institutions' news release
*Reference: Shim H, Dang C, Proceedings of the National Academy of Sciences USA, 1998 Feb 17; 95(4): 1511-1516.

ON CARDIOVASCULAR DISEASE:

'Hence, many observations indicating reductions in plasma lipid levels when people are on low-fat diets may be due to changes I the fatty acid composition of the diet, not the reduction of fat calories.'

*Reference: Nelson, GJ, et al, Lipids, 'Low-Fat Diets do not Lower Plasma Cholesterol Levels in Healthy Men Compared to High-Fat Diet With Similar Fatty Acid Composition at Constant Caloric Intake' 1995Nov; 30(11): 969-76.

All cells have a coating of fat to protect them. Each cell has memory and if undamaged can repair itself easily.

The Framlington study

'In Framingham, Mass, the more saturated fat one ate, the more cholesterol one ate. The more calories one ate, the lower the person's serum cholesterol, we *found that the people who ate the most cholesterol, ate the most saturated fat, ate the most calories* weighed the least and were the most physically active.'

*Reference: Castelli, William, Archives of Internal Medicine, 1992 Jul; 152(7): 1371-1372

 (Serum cholesterol is blood cholesterol, and all hormones are made from this. It is not the same food cholesterol).

'Abnormalities in glucose and insulin metabolism are commonly found in patients with high blood pressure [1-9]'& 'there is evidence suggesting that defects in glucose and insulin metabolism may play a role in both the origin and the natural history of high blood pressure.'

*Reference: Reaven G. et al, The American Journal of Medicine 1989; 87(supp 6A):6A-2S

'If, as we had been told, heart disease results from the excesses of the consumption of saturated fats, one would expect to find a correspondingly large increase in animal fat in the American diet. Actually the reverse is true.

During the sixty year period from 1910 to 1970, the proportion of traditional animal fat in the American diet plummeted from 83% to 62%, the proportion of butter consumption from 18 pounds per person per year to 4. During the past eighty years dietary vegetable fat in the form of margarine, shortening and refined oils increase about 400% and the consumption of sugar and processed foods increase about 60%.

* Sally Fallon, Nourishing Traditions 1995 Promotion Publishing

*Reference: US Department of Agriculture statistics quoted in Douglass, William Campbell, MD The Milk of Human Kindness is Not Pasteurised, 1985 Copple House Books, Lakemont, Georgia, 184; and in Beasley, Joseph D, MD and Jerry J Swift, MA The Kellogg Report, 1989 The Institute of Health Policy and Practice, Annandale-on-Hudson, New York, 144.

'In the United States, 315 of every 100,000 middle aged men die of heart attacks each year; in France the rate is 145 per 100,000. In the Gascony region, where goose and duck liver form a staple of the diet, this rate is a remarkably low 80 per 100,000.'

* Sally Fallon, Nourishing Traditions 1995 Promotion Publishing

*Reference: The New York Times, November 17, 1991

'More plagues than heart disease can be laid at sugar's door. A survey of medical journals in the 1970's produced findings that implicated sugar as a causative factor in kidney disease, liver disease, shortened life-span, increased desire for coffee and tobacco, as well as arteriosclerosis and coronary heart disease.'
*Sally Fallon, Nourishing Traditions 1995 Promotion Publishing
*Reference: Howell, Edward, MD Enzyme Nutrition 1985 Avery Publishing Group, Inc

'Medical Research Council survey showed that men eating butter ran half the risk of developing heart disease as those using margarine.'
*Sally Fallon, Nourishing Traditions 1995 Promotion Publishing
*Reference: Nutrition Week March 22, 1991 21:12:2-3

ON DIABETES:

'A very high-fat, low-carbohydrate diet has been shown to have astounding effects in helping type 2 diabetics lose weight and improve their blood lipid profiles. . The thing many diabetics coming into the office don't realize is that other forms of carbohydrates will increase their sugar, too. Dieticians will point toward complex carbohydrates & oatmeal and whole wheat bread, but we have to deliver the message that these are carbohydrates that increase blood sugars, too.'

'These results suggest that a high protein, low-carbohydrate diet, with nutritional supplementation can be useful to reduce several cardiovascular risk factors in obese adult onset diabetic patients including weight, blood sugar, and lipid parameters.

24

There is also no evidence that the nutritional regimen adversely affects kidney function.'

*Reference: Edman, JS et al. Journal of the American College of Nutrition, to be published in October 1998.

'It seems prudent to avoid the use of low-fat, high-carbohydrate diets containing moderate amounts of sucrose in patients with non-insulin-dependent diabetes mellitus.'

*Reference: Coulston, A.M. et al, American Journal of Medicine 1987 Feb; 82(2):213-220.

'As compared with the high-carbohydrate diet, the High-monounsaturated-fat diet resulted in lower mean plasma glucose levels and reduced insulin requirements, lower levels of plasma triglycerides and very low-density lipo-protein cholesterol, and higher levels of high-density lipoprotein (HDL) (good) cholesterol. Levels of total cholesterol did not differ significantly in patients on the two diets.'

*Reference: Garg, A. et. al, New England Journal of Medicine 1988; 319 (13): 829-341.

ON STROKE:

'Intakes of fat, saturated fat, and monosaturated fat were associated with reduced risk of ischemic stroke in men.'(design and setting from the Framingham Heart Study).

*Reference: Gillman M. et al, Journal of the American Medical Association, 1997; 78(24): 2145-2150

ON THE LOW-FAT DIET:

'Low-fat diets - low in polyunsaturated fatty acids induce essential fatty acid (EFA) insufficiency, and can increase the biochemical risk factors for heart disease: they may also increase appetite.'

*Reference: Siguel, E. BioMedicina, January 1998; 1(1): 9 'low-fat, high carbohydrate diets also reduce high-density lipoprotein (HDL) cholesterol levels and raise fasting levels of triglycerides.'
*Reference: Mensink RP, et al, Arteriorscler Thromb 1992 Aug;12(8): 911-919

(They are called essential fatty acids because we die without them)

'Hence, many earlier observations indicating reductions in plasma lipid levels when people are on low-fat diets may be due to changes in the fatty acid composition of the diet, not the reduction calories.'

*Reference: Nelson, G.J. et al., Lipids 1995; 30(11): 969-976.

'The relative good health of the Japanese, who have the longest life-span in the world, is generally attributed to a low-fat diet'& those who point to Japanese statistics to promote the low-fat diet fail to mention that the Swiss live almost as long on one of the fattiest diets in the world. Tied for third in the longevity are Austria and Greece. Both with high fat diets.'

Sally Fallon, Nourishing Traditions 1995 Promotion Publishing

*Reference: Moore, Thomas J Lifespan: What Really Affects Human Longevity, 1990 Simon & Schuster, New York

'Mother's milk contains a higher portion of cholesterol than almost any other food. It also contains over 50% of its calories as fat, much of it saturated fat. Both cholesterol and saturated fat are essential for growth in babies and children, especially development of the brain. Yet the American Heart Association is now recommending a low-cholesterol, low-fat diet for children!'

Sally Fallon, Nourishing Traditions 1995 Promotion Publishing

*Reference: Alfin-Slater, RB and L Aftergood, 'Lipids', Modern Nutrition in Health and Disease, Chapter 5, 6th ed, RS Goodhart and ME Shils, eds, Lea and Febiger, Philadelphia 1980, p. 31

'There is still the potential for low-fat intakes to adversely affect the nutritional adequacy of the diet of children and Given the assumption that there are some potential nutritional dangers associated with the unsupervised use of such diets, with no proven benefits, this diet should definitely not be advocated for infants and young children.' *Reference: Zlotkin, SH Arch Pediatr Adolesc Med. 1997;151:962-963

'In 1821 the average sugar intake in America was 10 pounds per person per year; today it is 170 pounds per person, over one fourth the average caloric intake. Another large fraction of all calories comes from refined flour and refined vegetable oils.'
*Sally Fallon, Nourishing Traditions 1995 Promotion Publishing
*Reference: Beasley, Joseph D, MD and Jerry J Swift, MA The Kellogg Report, 1989 The Institute of Health Policy and Practice, Annandale-on-Hudson, New York, 144-145

The next chapter tells how – stage by stage – to set the healing process in motion. It is a six week course and it does need to be followed to the letter. Once you are well you can deviate a little from time to time, but by helping you to understand how important eating the right foods for YOU can take some grasping. Those who stick to the diet improve dramatically, weight and years slip away. Smiles and life comes back. I have seen hugely improved wellness happen just by changing the foods alone.

MORROR IMAGE

IS THIS YOU?

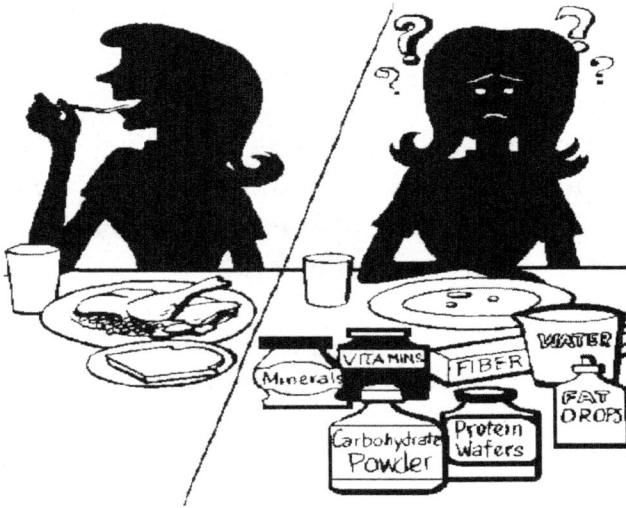

CAN'T DECIDE WHAT TO EAT AND WHAT NOT TO?
Start with shopping for the correct foods for all the family.

THE SIX WEEK PROTOCOL

A. Planning is the key to success. Spend time taking care to plan your next 6 weeks. Decide what changes you will make and how you will have the strength to carry those forward.

B. Learn how to write everything down in a journal. Keep a list of your weekly goals, what target are you aiming for?

C. Take the time to do this for yourself. There's no point in rushing and getting in a muddle. Start when the time is right for you.

D. Understand that food is NOT the only way to loose weight. It is a combination of lifestyle and being healthy in mind, body, and spirit.

E. Do follow your plan step by step; if you miss anything out go back to the beginning. It is important to get it right, even if this means going over and over until you have learnt it by heart.

F. Learn how to read labels. Even better do not buy anything with labels on them. If it's made in a factory then there's a high risk it has too many chemicals.

G. Learn how to plan your shopping. This is one of the most important aspects of weight loss. Temptation at the checkout and impulse buying is only human nature. However once the detox is completed do have one treat a week.

H. Adjust your mental attitude to positive, and be filled with hope. It is so important to want to be healthy and meditation can be a good starting point.

I. Make sure you do not have any bad influences around you. Loved ones sometimes like what they have, and often can feel threatened by change

J. One of the best things you can do is to remember that good quality water heals – but not tap or filtered water

K. Decide which exercise is best for you – be focused enough to do fifteen to 30 minutes each day.

L. Organise your life into healing mode.

M. Slowly start sleeping for eight hours a night it is important for healing, 9 hours is better, go to bed before midnight.

N. Buy a tape measure, jotter/notebook, thermometer, and pencil.

O. Affirmations do work – give them a try.

P Remember faith heals faster than anything.

Q. Stick to the foods you tested best for.

R. Remember it is not only for six weeks – but a diet for life. It's better to lose 3 lbs a week for a year than a stone in a month.

The next chapter deals with these points individually

CHAPTER FOUR

A. PLANNING

Discover time management. Divide up your week and days and hours into these categories:

1. work
2. leisure
3. sleeping
4. exercise
5. cooking/eating
6. meditation

A typical day should read:

Take temperature before rising, under arm with a glass thermometer for ten minutes, 98.4F 37C are normal.

8.00 am – rise take homeopathic medicine
   15 minutes exercise, (this can be done in bed)
   cook and eat breakfast
   shower/bath, get dressed
   work or however you fill your day

10.00 – eat and drink something go out into fresh air for five minutes (walk if possible)

12.30– lunch (prepared the night before, or at home)

3.00 – fruit or snack, drink, fresh air

(Blood sugar often dips around this time)
5.30 – walk for ten minutes

6.30 – dinner

The evening is for leisure (not in the pub).
Before bedtime – use meditation and yoga breathing
exercises for five minutes

10.30 – go to bed write a brief journal of signs and
symptoms, foods and how your day worked out.

Check your pottering about pulse it should be around 80-84
beats per minute. Do check for the whole minute.

THE JOURNAL

Keep a journal – e.g. temperature, pulse (pottering about),
foods, signs, and symptoms, sleeping pattern, work,
allergies etc. You can see a difference before and after if
you do the six week protocol.

EXAMPLES OF A JOURNAL

1] WEIGH YOURSELF ONCE A WEEK (in the same
spot, naked, before eating and drinking, but after using the
toilet).

2] MEASURE TEN POINTS OF YOUR BODY AT
WEIGH IN TIME – NECK, UPPER ARM, BUST/CHEST,
UNDER BUST, WAIST, BELLY BUTTON,
WIDEST/BUM, UPPER THIGH, ABOVE KNEE, CALF

3] WRITE DOWN ALL VITAMINS/SUPPLEMENTS.MEDICINES

4] WRITE DOWN SIGNS AND SYMPTOMS

5] WRITE DOWN EXERCISE – WHEN IT IS DONE

6] KEEP A NOTE OF TEMPERATURE (ON WAKING) AND PULSE

7] WRITE DOWN FOODS EATEN AND DRINKS CONSUMED

8] KEEP A NOTE OF ANY OUTSIDE INFLUENCES – SUCH AS STRESS AT WORK OR HOME ETC.

USE THIS AS A GUIDE TO HEALING FOR THE SIX WEEK PROTOCOL

You will see clearly how you have improved over the six weeks. Weight loss of around five pounds is the most common loss in a week. BUT your measurements will reduce and clothes should fit better.

Your under arm temperature should also improve, medicine and supplements need to be in balance for this.

Measure and weigh yourself once or twice a week at the most.

Split the page of your journal into sections:

1. weight and measurements
2. signs and symptoms
3. how you feel

<u>TAKING TIME FOR YOURSELF</u>

Design your day so that you do things for yourself. These could include many things like having a nap or perhaps aromatherapy. Take care of yourself.

Close your eyes and imagine you are a small child again. Look after yourself as well as you should when you are little. For example you would not smoke as a child; so do not do it as an adult. You would not drink as a child; so do not do it. You would go to bed early as a child – perhaps reading before going to sleep. You would eat regularly and love life. Do not lose this child within, if it dies then so can your inner spirit.

Reading current publications about health is both a good thing. Do it but not at bedtime. Fill your mind with pleasant things and watching horror movies is not advised.

You should always allow some time for yourself in each day. Make your own space. Make those around you understand that you need to be alone at times to clear your mind.

As time goes on you will adjust, lose your food and emotional cravings, and begin to feel healthier.

FOOD IS NOT THE ONLY WAY TO LOOSE WEIGHT

You need to allow time for exercise; small amounts each day are needed. Ten to fifteen minutes in the morning will boost your metabolism and relax you. Exercise gives off endorphins – pleasure hormones in the brain. Simple stretching also helps.

You need to raise your metabolism. The three most common ways to do this are: exercise, diet, and lifestyle. They simply should not be stressed in any way.

Your environment is also vital. If you partner and or family or boss are in conflict this creates stress which inflates those delicate stress hormones of the adrenals. Constant stress reduces DHEA the balancing hormone.

If you consider what happens to the body when hydrocortisone, and/or Deltacortril (cortisol) is introduced artificially – swollen tummy and weight gain are one result. These are stress hormones. However if these are the opposite and too low then thyroid metabolism can be reduced. These two hormones work in harmony at a cellular level.

Find a way to sort out your problems without shouting or arguing, and if it is that bad walk away. Read some of the many self help books around.

The bottom line is that unhappiness = weight problems.

Be positive and you will become stronger as time goes on. Life can be an addiction itself. Addiction comes in many forms from abuse to laziness.

REMEMBER SHOPPING CAN BE FUN!

If it is on the list put it in your trolley – if not don't

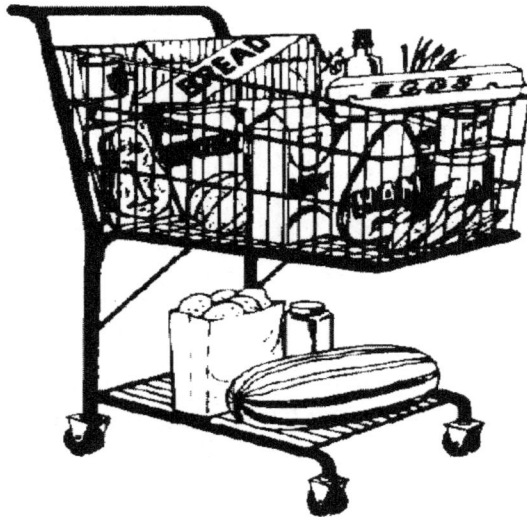

SHOP FOR HEALTH

HOW TO READ LABELS

Colorings - E102, 104, 110, 162, 150 is caramel. E127 is a stimulant and now banned as a food coloring, however it can be found in imported foods such as French glace cherries.

These are found in processed food, squash, soft drinks, jam, margarine, biscuits and cakes. They are asthma and hyperactivity triggers. Avoid.

E - numbers generally - E412, 414, 440, 460, 322, 422 are found in sauces, soups, bread, biscuits, cakes, desserts, ice cream, margarine, spreads, jam, chocolate, milk shakes. They can cause flatulence.

Avoid **Flavorings** - MSG, (monosodiumglutomate), 621, 622, 631. Found in Chinese food, gravy powders, stock cubes, packet soups, tinned and processed meat. MSG is a thyroid inhibitor and in large doses gives hallucinations. Avoid.

Lecithin – is known as E322. Prevalent in chocolate. It is a protein and a hormone released by fat travels in blood to the brain. Lecithin means thin. The more fat that you have the more lecithin is produced. It acts on the hypothalamus where it inhibits the amount of food we eat. It stops us from being hungry and limits energy expenditure by a signal to the hypothalamus.

Preservatives - Nitrates are E249-52 found in processed meat and smoked fish. Benzoates are E249-19 found in soft drinks, beer and salad cream.

Sulphates are E220-28 found in dried fruit, desiccated coconut, and relishes. Antioxidants are E300-304 found in fruit juice, jam, and tinned fruit. E320-21 are found in crisps, biscuits and pies. These E numbers are asthma triggers. Avoid.

Sorbitol, Aspartame and sweeteners all affect the anterior pituitary. Canned drinks, some yoghurts, milk drinks, and sweets are the worst. Sorbitol is also a laxative.

Obviously if the label contains a food or product you are toxic to avoid it too.

Don't listen to anyone else when it comes to food. The food industry is amazing at getting us to buy their products. It was the food industry in California that came up with the 5 a day is best for you. It was all advertising to sell more fruit and vegetables and had little to do with research.

PLANNING THE SHOPPING

1. write a list before you leave home
2. shop on your own
3. order shopping over the phone if you are short of time
4. shop organic
5. make time to do this without being rushed
6. do not shop when you are hungry
7. stick to the good foods
8. stick to the budget
9. don't shop if you are tired or stressed

ADJUST YOUR MENTAL ATTITUDE

The power of the mind is far greater than we give it credit for. Healing yourself should be top of your important list.

You can think yourself healthy. The Louise Hay books are very positive in their advice for mental healing. An example for overweight is:
Fear, running away from feelings, insecurity, self rejection

The affirmation is:

"I am at peace with my own feelings. I am safe. I create my own security. I love myself".

If you don't have someone to love – love yourself at least.

The voice in our heads often needs to be reprogrammed. Remember mental thoughts are electricity and energy. Thoughts should be good and pure. Anger destroys and drains. Be calm, be sweet, and be nice. If it's negative take it out of your head.

Replace all old patterns of thought like resentment, guilt etc.

Make a cosmic wish list. Examples are (in past tense always):
"I am happy, my life is wonderful, I am slim, and I love myself".

Put the past behind you and learn from it. It is in the past so leave it there. That includes your old thoughts. Start afresh. Think of your body as your friend.

Open your mind and do not be limited in your aspirations.

Discover what personality type you are. Example type A's are dominant, urgent people, these have less arterial damage and lower cholesterol levels.

Be in control of yourself.

BAD INFLUENCES

What are bad influences?
1. yourself and that devil that sits on your shoulder
2. your partner
3. your family
4. your friends
5. advertising
6. television
7. radio
8. magazines
9. newspapers

Take out and resist any negative brainwashing from the above. Ask do they have the same goals for me to be well as I do? If not ask why do they feel that way. Make sure this is what they want too!

HEALING WATER

We are 70% water. Water in its' natural form mimics the blood exactly. Molecule for molecule blood and water are the same.

When water travels for miles along iron or plastic pipes it changes composition. Filtering water does not put it back into its original state. Osmosis (imploding) can restructure somewhat.

Our tap water is so poisonous to our natural states. Outbreaks of Legionnaires Disease in Europe sent our chlorine levels up to double.

Tap water contains parasites like cryptosporidium, washed down from the water table of the land. The parasite gives tummy cramps, wind, gas and the trots.

We need six large glasses per day to make hormones, and clean our kidneys and body of toxins. It is very good for you with the odd squeeze of natural lemon juice.

Avoid fluoridated water at all costs. It will stop the thyroid working and may also give you acne. Also avoid fluoride in toothpaste.

Fluoride is more toxic than most poisons.

EXERCISE

There are so many exercise videos, books, and programmes. Choose one that fits you. One that is simple and straightforward. One that you can learn to do with your eyes closed if need be.

Are you blood group 'O'? They need to exercise – and a lot - especially walking.

Blood group 'A' people are usually gentle souls preferring yoga, stretching and rambling.

Blood group 'B's can be either lazy or frantic exercisers.

Blood group 'AB's are a combination of all the above.

1. stretching – slow and gentle, you can even do this in the chair or bed
2. yoga – the most complete exercise as it exercises the mind too
3. any walking – the adrenal glands are also exercised by walking. The valve in the calf pumps the blood back up to the heart. Begin slowly and build up. Use either a pedometer or your watch.
4. swimming – in moderation because of the chlorine
5. aerobics can be added to the exercise routine if your heart is not sick, leave until later in the six week programme
6. golf is good as it combines stretching and walking, remember to warm up first

7. any relaxation exercise before sleep; tighten toes, then feet and gradually work up the body tightening and relaxing slowly.

You should do some exercise each day even if just for five minutes. Start slowly and gradually build up is best. Walking increases the metabolism. Light jogging is only recommended in the fifth week.

Starting to exercise:

While warm in bed do some exercises, this is especially recommended for those who have weak backs. Build up to 10 sets of 100, you can do arm exercises while doing buttock squeezes. Design your own regime. Start slowly and build up.

Later in the day, lunchtime is best for maximum sunshine, unless you live in a really hot climate, walk for 20 minutes.

HEALING THOUGHTS

Think yourself well. Meditate in peace (no TV, radio etc.) have silence if possible. Meditation is calming, healing, strengthening. There are many books on meditation but it is easy to concentrate on a colour or image – keep out those negative thoughts. Chant if you want – use a healing affirmation. Use calm music if this helps you. Start with a colour – say – blue your mind may move naturally to the sea or sky, imagine a gentle sea or sky. Try to avoid all violent and or aggressive thoughts. Blue is the colour of the thyroid. Learn the chakra colours; add these healing colours to your décor in the home and work.

Colour therapy is one of the easiest to do yourself; it can be as easy as doing a simple water colour. Some people are drawn to primary colours, look at your environment, and see what colours you surround yourself with. Also what colours do you wear most often and ask yourself why you are drawn to them.

When you practice meditation on a regular basis you will be able to put a ring of calmness around yourself.

Remember fate takes us in many directions and on many roads in our lifetime. They are for a purpose. Adversity can be overcome – be strong.

SLEEPING

Most hypothyroids have bizarre sleeping patterns. They go to bed and cannot go to sleep – heart pounding, brain whizzing around. They when it is time for the average person to wake up most are just entering their deep sleeping pattern. Most don't see breakfast for many years. It's common to fall asleep or go through phases of sleeping in the afternoon and or at teatime. If you need to sleep to top up your hormones then do it in a safe place.

The Bedroom

1. do not have it too hot or cold
2. wear clothing to keep you warm
3. don't feel guilty about having a hot water bottle
4. make sure the air in the bedroom is changed each day – open a window

5. sleep only on a single pillow – hypo-allergenic is best as it curves to the shape of your head (if you are not allergic to it)
6. do not leave the central heating on all night, running water affects the body's energy patterns
7. make sure the room is warm enough using insulation
8. do not have any electricity near your head
9. beds pointing north give the best nights sleep
10. do not have a wireless connection or mobile phone on in the room

Be calm when you go to bed. If you have problems regulating your sleeping try ordering melatonin from USA. DO NOT TAKE sleeping tablets; sleeping should be as natural as possible.

If your thyroid is too low you will probably snore. If it is too low you will not go into deep REM healing sleep. Snoring is a good indicator of low thyroid function

Hormones are made when you sleep. If your hormones are too low you will feel exhausted. If you sleep normally when you wake up your hormone levels are at their highest.

Try to organise sleeping by exercise, foods, hormones, and lifestyle. You will once again have a simple sleeping pattern; it does come back in time.

Calcium tablets and or milk help sleeping. If your calcium is too low you may have sleeping problems.

Lavender oil on your pillow or on your feet will help sleeping.

Sex can both help and stop sleeping – many of you may have lost your sex drive and given it up but it does sometimes help.

Noise pollution is one of the worst things for those light hypothyroid sleepers. People with thyroid problems are usually sensitive to noise. Adding blackout blinds or shutters to a room can help.

If you wake up, and feel to hot then do take your under arm temperature. You may see that you are actually too cold. It may be time to check your thyroid supplements to see if the dose is high enough.

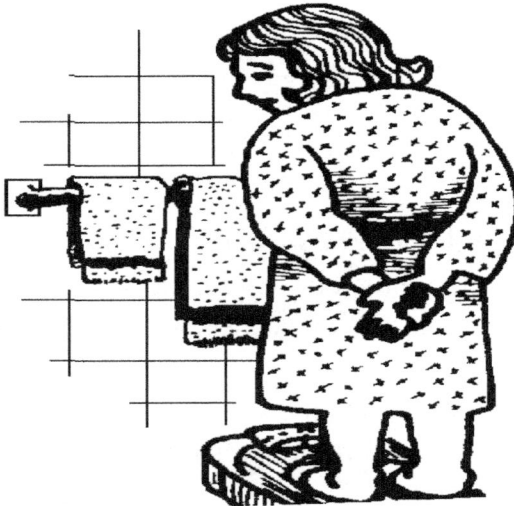

SHE REALLY SHOULD BE NAKED

CHAPTER FIVE

THE TOOLS TO HEAL

This is a list of books and items you will need to loose weight;
Dr. Atkins – Age-defying Diet
Dr. Atkins – New Diet
Louisa Hay – any of them
Naomi Ozaniec – Beginners Guide to Dowsing
Dr. Peter D' Adamo – Eat Right Diet (for your blood group)

Jotter for a journal

Tape measure for those ten points

Scales for weight – remember muscle weighs heavier than fat

Pencil for jotter

Pedometer/watch for walking

Shopping list for foods

Diary for time management

Thermometer for under arm temperature

Take a photo before and after of your face and full body.

MENUS

Breakfast
Eggs, bacon, fish, fruit, yoghurt, fresh juice, (from Dr. Atkins' list)

10.30
Fruit, berries are best or natural bio-yoghurt, mineral water, fresh juice

Lunch
Meat and fruit or salad water/herb tea

Afternoon
Fruit, mineral water, nuts, fresh juice

Dinner
Meat (fish) and vegetables (not cabbage, sprouts, greens, turnip or cruciferous) juice, water

Night – spring water and 2 sea calcium or coral calcium tablets

(Calcium is one of the lowest minerals in our bodies. Check iron - also an indicator or low thyroid and Vitamin D).

While detoxing use CoQ10 (1 x 30 mg) and psyllium hulls (2 at night) to help remove the dead parasites from your system.

THE NO LIST

Starchy foods, bread, pasta, peanuts, biscuits, some high sugar over ripe fruits (banana), rice, rice cakes, excess of dairy foods, potatoes, all alcohol. All carbonated drinks. All citrus juices, they are too acid. Wine, beer a d fermented items like hard cheese, yeast etc.

Aluminium cooking pots and foil in any form.

THE YES LIST IS EVERYTHING YOUR TEST SHOWS YOU BALANCE WITH, THESE COULD BE:
Nuts, fish (careful many people are toxic to it), fruits, vegetables (not cabbage family), salads, meat, pure virgin olive oil, eggs, butter, cream (in moderate amounts).

If you have aching joints and or arthritis avoid all the nightshade family – these are potatoes, tomatoes, peppers, aubergines (egg plant)

Eczema can be linked to poor liver function, chemicals and a worm. Alcohol should be avoided inside but a 50/50 dilute of vodka and water dabbed into the site often help. Also try avoiding dairy products. This distressing illness can be caused by food allergies.

If you are sick and tired of being sick and tired you will stick to the protocol which includes foods, vitamins, and correct supplements, conventional and homeopathic medicine.

Do not overdo the supplements. It's better to be tested for what you need, and even better to get those from food. Too many are as bad as too little. Be tested first and as you begin to change your diet your need for excessive supplement taking should reduce as the six week protocol ends.

An example of a journal would include most of the items listed below:

Weight (weekly)   Temperature (upon waking) daily

Pulse not aerobic or resting

Medicine - make sure the dose is correct

Vitamins   do you need them?

Supplements, these can be natural

Measurements: do weekly but not before menstruation.

Foods: daily foods eaten   Drinks: all consumed daily

Signs and symptoms: It is important to do these on a regular basis as you will see that as you progress and are on the correct protocol your healing will show in your notes.

Sleeping times: The go to bed time, and the time it takes you to go to sleep.

Waking times: do you wake up through the night, can you go right back to sleep. Do you get up and watch TV?

Worst feeling: (emotions) how do these improve? When the swollen tummy subsides does it have a positive effect on you?

Stressors: what upset you and why did you let it upset you?

PERFECT _BALANCE FOR HEALING_

1. have your lymph balanced
2. have your foods, vitamins and supplements tested for allergy and intolerance
3. organise your life
4. be happy
5. exercise daily in small amounts, 15 minutes walking in a green place is best
6. sleep well, more than 8 hours
7. enjoy your life
8. be brave about your expectations
9. by healing and cleansing your gut you will have more energy
10. by healing your mind your stress levels will fall
11. weight is a heavy burden a positive approach is needed
12. have support from your loved ones – if you feel you will suffer ridicule keep the protocol to yourself
13. eat organic and local where possible
14. don't buy foods not on your balanced list
15. do take homeopathic medicine
16. do take your supplements, digestive enzymes and vitamins in which you are lacking
17. have faith in yourself
18. always do keep a record of how you feel, what you measure etc.
19. remember the six week protocol is for YOU and no one else – do not inflict your diet upon others unless they are tested too
20. call for advice if you have any problems
21. do the bowel cleanse first
22. do the detox with the bowel cleanse
23. keep a record of your temperature and pulse daily

Remember the Hunzas live in the extreme northern point of India. They walk 10 miles daily, do not give up work, eat simple foods – chicken is their source of protein. They live a stress free life. Disease is unknown. Remember the word disease means the body is not at ease.

The father of modern medicine was Hypocrites. He lived over 2000 years ago in Greece. His basic approach is that food is your best medicine. Or you are what you eat. The Hunzas get up at five, go to bed early, and eat only two meals a day. Their diet is a mixture of fruits, vegetables, chicken, and yoghurt. Old is a state of mind. Keep that child within – reset your inner timepiece. Remember to breathe deeply thirty times each day in a fresh air place. Or try 15 twice a day.

To slim you need supplements to help you clean out and start with a clean gut. Remember most people loose 10lbs in six weeks on this diet; some have lost six pounds in a week. The most lost was 32lbs in five weeks.

WEIGHT LOSS PROGRAMME SIMPLIFIED 26 golden rules

1. Walking everyday, for 15 minutes out and 15 back, in a green or fresh air place, especially before 10:00 am. A lack of sunlight is implicated in MS. We need one hour of sunlight on our skins daily for vitamin D. This should also increase bone density. Walking stimulates our adrenal glands; the point for these is on the ball of the foot. Use flat base trainers. Also add in stretching and bed exercises.

2. Going to bed before 10:00 pm lowers cortisol the stress hormone. Also, in deep sleep is where HGH, human growth hormone, is released. HGH regulates our body mass. That is why you should feel so refreshed and in good shape after a good night sleep (among other reasons, of course). Wheat reduces cortisol, causing sleeping problems. Walking for 10 minutes before bedtime helps sleeping.

3. 8 small glasses of boiled/cooled spring water per day (fluoride free and low in nitrates) - a cup an hour. Add fresh lemon juice for cleansing. Bicarbonate of soda or calcium will alkalize the stomach. ¼ teaspoon of cider vinegar for acid

problems and candida. Acidy tummy can also mean calcium is too low.

4.   No refined carbohydrates, low complex carbohydrates only from vegetables and fruits. Limit/exclude grains, no gluten - it inhibits absorption of nutrients by coating the digestive system with glue. 100 grams of good quality protein per day, the protein in grains interferes with thyroid proteins.

5.   At least 3 fluid ounces of high quality fats and oils throughout the day. Essential fatty acids are called this because we die and age without them. For fish oil - be sure it is heavy metal, mercury, and hexane free. Protein and fat equal new healthy cells. Fats and oils help with the body's communications on all levels and everything is improved by increasing them. Half a cup of oils, (not a mug,) and fats each day. Oily fish at least once a week.

6.   5 – 6 cups of a variety of vegetables each day, not regular potatoes. 5 brands of vegetables and fruit per day. Berries open up blood vessels and are anti-oxidants.

7.   Some form of gentle weight lifting with just 5 lbs is good enough. You just need to be regular with it - at least 3 times per week x 20 minutes.

8.   You should aim at a gradual weight loss and it can happen by increasing the good things, and decreasing the not so good gradually. The first week your loss should be around half a stone then 2 – 3 lbs each week thereafter. Muscle weighs heavier than fat. Measure 10 points of your body once a week. Remember to weigh yourself in the morning, naked once a week.

9.   Affirmations work incredibly well - for instance, "Everyday in every way I feel better and better." Be happy, say "I feel happy and slim" regularly – out loud.

10. Stand up tall. Posture is vital, do not slouch. Use yoga stretching for a perfectly toned body.

11. Do a complete detox before you start your diet, this should be: a] parasite cleanse, 2] kidney cleanse, 3] liver cleanse, 1 week gap then repeat. You can have 2 – 3 stones of parasites living in you. This may make you tired at first. You can also have a headache for a couple of days.

12. Obey the rules of the stomach. Always be allergy, food, mineral, hormone, and nutrition tested. Do not drink after meals. Drink half a pint before eating and just have a couple of mouthfuls after eating to wash out your gullet.

13. A body that is slightly alkaline cannot get ill, Avoid acid foods like grains and nightshade. Do not eat white coloured foods, except eggs.

14. Always be allergy/intolerance tested for foods before beginning any diet. Eat breakfast and 3 good meals per day. Snack on fruit/nuts.

15. Avoid toxic items like caffeine, alcohol, smoking, processed foods and drinks.

16. Cook only at moderate temperature. Micro-waving kills 70 – 80% of enzymes. Never microwave anything. Do not use aluminium either for cooking or foil. Keep metals to a minimum. Cook in spring water or rain-water.

17. Do not buy processed/industrial food. Cook it yourself from local fresh produce.

18. What you give out you get back, being negative gets negative. Reap and sow good thoughts and emotions.

19. We are what we eat and how we feel. The things that make us ill are trauma, pollution, and parasites.

20. Use an EMF screener and keep electricity away from you while sleeping. Your bedroom should be a sanctuary.

21. Keep chemicals away from you and your environment. Use only natural products and clothing if you can afford it.

22. What fills your life expands. If that is food then you will eat and want more.

23. Use small cutlery, plates, and bowls. The crockery you eat off should not be bigger than your hand finger tips to wrist.

24. If you wouldn't do or give it a 3 year old then do not do it or give it to yourself.

25. Be kind to yourself.

26. Once a week eat and drink what you want.

27. Don't give up.

THREE PARTS OF NUTRITION

1. There are some basic essential elements of nutrition that have been misunderstood and lacking in our diets.

2. We know the need for vitamins, enzymes, and co-enzymes factors that allow for the development of energy, neurological function and other factors of life.

3. We also know our need for protein, but actually protein is broken up in the digestive system and what our body really needs are amino acids.

4. What we don't realize is our need for fatty acids. Fatty acids are building blocks for cell membranes. These fatty acids and many of the amino

acids are heat liable and are destroyed by over cooking. In our society, over cooking and processing of our foods is very common.

5.   A three-part program was developed to supply the body with these basic elements of nutrition. 1) *FATTY ACIDS supply the essential fatty acids for health, 2) *AMINO ACIDS supplies the basic amino acids and minerals for health, and 3) *A-Z VITAMIN supplies the vitamins and coenzyme factors needed for health.

6.   Fatty acids, amino acids and minerals, and vitamins are the key ingredients that are often missing in our present diet due to overcooking and processing of foods. With good simple nutrition and these additional products, nutritional balancing can occur. This allows for an increase in health and maximizes the body's ability to cure itself.

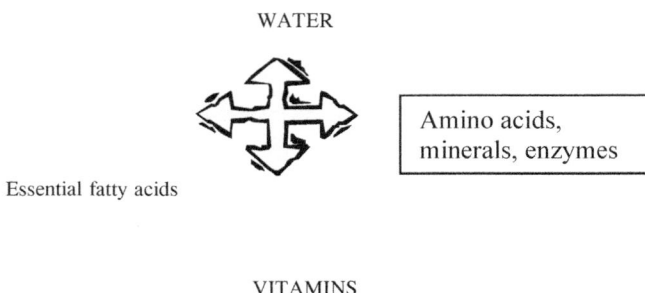

WATER

Essential fatty acids

Amino acids, minerals, enzymes

VITAMINS

THYROID METABOLISM

The thyroid is a highly important gland in the neck that regulates metabolism, among a vast array of other things. There are over 500 different functions related to the thyroid gland that are known by current medical science; there may be more that are not known.

Dr. Broda Barnes believed that 40 - 45% of the population was hypothyroid, and had a problem with not making enough of the thyroid hormone. This hypothyroid condition could lead to headaches and many other diseases. Dr. Barnes felt that brain swelling, caused by low-thyroid function, was responsible for

56

many migraine attacks. Depression was related to hypothyroidism, as without the metabolism hormone of the thyroid, the person would feel sluggish, lethargic, and depressed. Chronic fatigue can result from Hypoadrenia (low adrenals) and hypothyroidism. The most common complaint is that of weakness or fatigue, which no amount of sleep seems to cure. Weight gain, bloating, and weight management all result from hypothyroidism.

Anaemia can sometimes be one of the results of low thyroid, as a hypothyroid can lead to under-active bone marrow, which cannot manufacture the quality and the quantity of red blood cells.

Sluggish digestion leads to digestive disturbances, which can also lead to anaemia and malnutrition syndrome.

Hypothyroid cases will tend to develop calluses on the feet. They will tend to be obese, tend to be cold, and chill easily; and tend to lack motivation. Thyroid Liquescence homeopathic can often help manage such disorders.

Hyperthyroid cases are those that tend to have over hot bodies, high metabolism, often "bug eyes" that stick out of the sockets, nervous disorders, inability to handle stress, tachycardia, heart irregularities. Usually low adrenals cause this. If the temperature is higher than 98.2, there might possibly be a hyperthyroid case, in which case vitamin A is an excellent anti-thyroid hormone. When combined with selenium and vitamin E, its effect is even greater, (sunflower oil).

The Barnes's test for hypothyroidism was to place a thermometer underneath the armpit for ten minutes, upon awakening in the morning. The temperature should read between 97.8 and 98.2. This is known as auxiliary body temperature. If the temperature reads below 97.8, and there is a significant health problem, it might be rectified or assisted to be cured by giving some thyroid hormone. This can be prescribed by the preventative-oriented physician.

It is possible to use food state natural thyroid and other hormones to control hyper and hypothyroid. This is not a cure and need to be taken regularly or the symptoms return. The daily dose varies slightly but on average 3 – 4 porcine extra strong natural thyroid and 5 – 6 bovine work best. For those who have low adrenals adrenal glandular often helps.

Other hormones that also help are: wild yam to balance female hormones, natural progesterone, DHEA, and pregnenolone for the over 50's. It's best to be tested to see what would work best to balance you and this can be done using the hair analysis. Your hair is like an imprint of the rest of you. It contains not only minerals, nutrition, and hormones but also emotions and everything in your aura energy field.

Getting the hormone balance is important for both metabolism and wellness. What suits one person may not suit another; we are all different in our emotions, hormones, life styles, and experiences. No one ever tested us when we felt well so there are no basic levels to refer to.

DIET FOR A HEALTHY LIFE

Unless you have food allergies the following diet is recommended: all should be organic where possible. *YOU SHOULD ALWAYS BE TESTED FIRST BEFORE EMBARKING ON ANY DIET. Not all foods are good for all people. What balances you will be different to another person because we are individuals and not clones of each other.*

Blackberries	any berries	Strawberries
Meat daily		Celery
Free range eggs max. Ten medium per week		Watercress
Herb teas		Cream

Minerals – calcium, zinc, magnesium, iron	Mango
Papaya	Carrots
Liver once per week	Berries
Lemons, they have perfect pH.	Peaches
Apples (washed + peeled).	Pineapple
Ginger	Apricots
Mushrooms (for B12)	
Dandelion, gooseberry	Bean sprouts
Spring water – (check mineral water for fluoride, nitrates, and sulphates.)	Yam
Glucose when energy levels are too low	Butter
Poultry whenever you feel like it.	Good oils
Bramley or cooking apples with honey	Parsley
Bananas twice per week	Elderberry
Grapes if washed thoroughly	Spinach
Red wine twice per week (one glass only – dilute with spring water)	
Sweet potatoes	Honey
Lettuce, (not iceberg)	Vegetable oil
Dill, rosemary, tarragon, fennel, basil, bay, sage	
Vegetables	Full Milk

FOODS FOR DAILY MENUS

The objectives of these recipes are to keep them simple, quick, easy to follow, to be nourishing, and to be balanced. Always prepare from fresh.

BREAKFAST

Eating Breakfast at Home

1) Rice bread toast with good quality butter
2) Rice flour pancakes with butter and lemon (natural), unsweetened home made apple sauce, or jam made with pure fruit (no honey or sugar)
3) One or two poached or boiled eggs with rice cake/rice toast and butter
4) Scrambled egg with mushrooms
5) Bacon, eggs, mushrooms and bean sprouts – or Any COMBINATION OF.

6) Edam or mozzarella cheese melted over rice bread fried in butter
7) Baked yam (cook it while you're dressing) with butter and cream cheese
8) Do-It-Yourself Protein Drink, liquidize any protein with either berries/milk or veg.
9) occasionally, unsweetened bio yogurt with fruit
10) Any combination of vegetables lightly fried in vegetable oil with meat

Eating Breakfast Out

1) Bacon and eggs
2) Omelette (spinach and mushroom, sautéed vegetable, ratatouille, Spanish)
3) Ham and vegetables
4) Fruit and cheese
5) Any vegetable combination with meat

RICE BREAD SQUARES

Toast 2 slices of rice bread (available in the organic section of the supermarket)
Thinly spread with butter
Layer with spinach (always soak in salt water first)
Cover in thin layers of mozzarella cheese
Grill until golden brown

EGGS AND BACON

Grill 2 rashers of bacon and then slice with scissors
Whisk 2 free-range eggs and one fluid oz. double cream together
Melt a knob of butter in a pan
Whisk the eggs until cooked   Add bacon and serve

QUICK HAM BREAKFAST

Sliced ham
Sliced mushrooms
Lightly fry together in ½ oz butter
Add bean sprouts

Toss together and serve

FRUIT SALAD

1 Mango cubed
1 small papaya cubed
1 passion fruit
Wash, peel, cube, add passion fruit and one fluid oz. double cream

CRUNCHY CORN PATTIES

Liquidise sweet corn with egg and a little cream or milk
Add rice flour to thicken
Form round patties
Lightly fry in butter until golden brown
Can be eaten with organic baked beans or cold

LUNCH

Eating Lunch at Home or Bringing It to Work

1) Salad with beans (pinto red, garbanzo) and rice cake and butter
2) Salad with a small amount of chicken, turkey, meat, egg
3) Salad with a full fat cheese (a nice occasional treat)
4) A hearty soup, like meat and bean, with a salad
5) Vegetables raw with chicken/meat grilled
6) Chicken breast and marinated vegetables
7) Steamed or sautéed vegetables with brown rice
8) Cold meat sliced over fresh vegetables/salad
9) Hummus (garbanzo bean dip) with rice cakes and salad
10) Hummus with raw vegetables
11) Raw vegetables soaked in sea salt and drained, juiced to make a drink
12) Occasionally, mozzarella cheese

Eating Lunch Out

1) Salad with egg, or chicken
2) Salad bar with bean salad and/or garbanzo beans, and juice
3) Chicken with salad or cooked vegetables
4) Chicken, turkey, or egg-salad
5) Soup and/or a salad
6) Chinese vegetables with chicken and a little rice (no MSG)
7) Vegetable omelette with a little cheese and spring rolls
8) Oily fish and simple vegetables
9) Steamed vegetables and any protein

DINNER

Eating Dinner at Home

1) Spicy Chinese Vegetables and chicken/meat
2) Sautéed vegetables with brown rice
3) Steamed vegetables with meat or brown rice
4) Vegetable soup with salad
5) Roasted meat and salad
6) Chicken breasts in cream sauce with vegetables
7) Chicken with salad or vegetables
8) Curried vegetables with tofu and brown rice
9) Vegetable soup with toasted rice bread
10) Corn tortillas – gluten free with beans and hot sauce (salsa) and salad
11) Rice bread and organic baked beans and side salad
12) Spanish rice with vegetables or salad
13) Steamed vegetables with meat and tomato sauce
14) Salad and baked sweet potato, sliced meat

Eating Dinner Out

1) Roasted meat/chicken with vegetables and salad
2) Chicken dishes with cream sauces on the side (use sparingly), with
      Vegetables and salad
3) Chinese food (no MSG) with chicken or bean curd (tofu) and a little rice
      (no pork, fish, or shrimp)
4) Italian food: veal, chicken, meat with salad and/or vegetables
5) Chicken enchilada or chicken tostada with cheese with salsa
6) Soup and salad

Snacks

1) Homemade soups (boil a chicken carcass and add vegetables)
2) Rice cakes, butter or mayo and meat/eggs/fish
3) Raw vegetables (soaked in sea salt to cleanse them first)
4) Small amounts of fruit, no bananas. Berries are best.
5) Salad in a bowl
6) Popcorn, natural
7) Cold sliced meat
8) Natural fruits
9) Plums
10) Nuts, not peanuts
11) Small pot natural yoghurt, you can add berries to this.
12) Only 2 bananas per week for healthy potassium levels.

The general guide to snacks is that you do not eat more than the amount that covers the palm of your hand.

MAIN MEALS

BROCCOLI, BACON AND CHEESE

1 Head of broccoli soaked in salt water
3 – 4 rashers of bacon
¼ pint of full fat milk
½ oz. butter
2 teaspoonfuls of corn flour
Pinch of parsley (optional)
1 oz. soft cheese, full fat
Pinch of sea salt

Lightly cook the broccoli
Fry or grill the bacon
Boil the milk and butter, add parsley and corn flour to thicken, add cheese
Snip bacon into small pieces, mix with broccoli, and cover with the sauce

COD/FISH PIE

Use 4 oz. of frozen fish, brush with oil
Place in a Pyrex dish and a medium oven and cook until flaky
Boil sliced carrots, broccoli, or beans until half cooked
Add to the fish
Cover with parsley sauce (as in recipe above)
Further cook for 5 minutes

CRISPY CORNED BEEF

Boil half a yam, and mash with black pepper and sea salt to taste
Pit 4 slices of corned beef into a Pyrex dish and cover with the mashed yam
Lightly brush with butter and grill until golden brown
Serve with fresh vegetables

BEEF IN MUSHROOM GRAVY

Make standard gravy by melting ½ oz butter with ¼ pint boiled spring water
and adding gravy powder
Put 4 slices of beef into a Pyrex dish and cover with 3 oz. mushrooms
Pour over the gravy
Slice sweet potatoes thinly and make a lid on the beef and mushrooms
Cook until sweet potatoes are crispy in a medium oven

LAMB AND MINT

2 Lamb chops or fillet of lamb
Place in a Pyrex dish
Cover with mint sauce (2 teaspoons)
Wash and scrub a sweet potato and bake alongside the lamb
Boil sliced runner beans and serve with butter

CHICKEN AND HONEY MUSTARD

Slice chicken breast and layer with mushrooms
Cover with ¼ pint of white sauce and ¼ teaspoon of honey mustard
Dice celeriac and/or yam into one-inch squares and boil until almost cooked
Drain yam and cover chicken add a few knobs of butter and grill until golden
brown

ROASTED VEGETABLES

Peel and cube the following vegetables:
2 parsnips
2 carrots
½ yam
2 sweet potatoes
Toss all in oil and place in Pyrex dish, sprinkle with sea salt and cook in a medium oven until golden brown

INDIAN CHICKEN

Remove the skin from 3 chicken drumsticks
Score the flesh both ways
Cover with a marinade of the following:
1 oz. bio yogurt (aspartame free)
1 oz. double cream
1 oz. balsamic vinegar
1 oz. oil
½ juice of a lemon
1 teaspoon of curry mix powder
Place in a Pyrex dish, cover with cling film and leave in fridge overnight
Remove the film and bake in a medium oven until brown
Slice sweet potatoes and toss in oil and lemon juice, cook until crispy
Serve with fresh basil/parsley and spinach tossed together

TURKEY SLICES

Place 3 slices of turkey breast in a Pyrex dish
Cream together: fresh basil, spinach, sultanas with 1fluid oz. double cream
Place mixture on the turkey and roll
Serve hot or cold

BEEF CASSEROLE

Cube ½ lb best beef, coat lightly in corn flour and fry in oil
Place in Pyrex dish
Add sliced carrots and 1 parsnip
Add spring water to cover and sea salt to taste
Slice yam and cover beef to form a lid
Cook until yam is crispy
Cover with standard gravy

SMOKED HADDOCK

Put 2 pieces of smoked haddock/fish from frozen into a Pyrex dish
Coved with spinach
Pour over a cream sauce
Serve with beans

CHICKEN AND PINEAPPLE

Melt a knob of butter in a frying pan
Add sliced chicken breast and cubed pineapple
Bring juice to boil and thicken with corn flour

Serve with mashed yam or bean sprouts

STEAMED VEGETABLES AND MEAT SAUCE

Dry fry the beef/meat
Add basic gravy and ¼ teaspoon of curry powder (optional)
Cook in medium oven
Steam any vegetables from the list
Pour the meat sauce over the vegetables

A BASIC SOUP

This can be added to with meat or extra vegetables, however it is delicious on its' own.

1 parsnip
1 sweet potato
2 medium carrots
½ oz. butter
Spring water to cover
Pinch sea salt
Boil until vegetables are soft and then mash

Alternatively boil up either a chicken carcass or some bones and use as a base stock. The stock can be frozen.

SALADS

PECAN AND CELERY SALAD

1 Celery heart, soak in salted water and slice thinly
Quarter pecan puts

Mix: 1oz. soft cheese
        1 tablespoon of full fat Hellmann's mayo
        1   "   double cream
Pour over. You can add to this, e.g. sultanas, nuts fresh pineapple

CRUNCHY SALAD

A handful of small spinach
A handful of lamb's lettuce
One celery heart finely sliced
½ a handful of sultanas
One fluid ounce of single cream mixed with one tablespoonful of Hellmann's mayo.

Lightly mix together

```
┌─────────────────────────────────────┐
│            DRESSING                  │
│                                      │
│  One fluid ounce of vinegar one      │
│  fluid ounce of oil                  │
│  A pinch of molasses sugar or        │
│  herbs to taste                      │
│  Sea salt                            │
│  Mix together                        │
└─────────────────────────────────────┘
```

BALSAMIC SALAD

2 oz. seedless grapes
2 oz. cashew nuts (unsalted)
Handful of lamb's lettuce
4 sticks of celery sliced

EGGS MAYONAISE

Slice 2 hard-boiled free-range eggs
Layer in a bowl with spinach or lambs lettuce

Dressing:

1 tsp tomato sauce
1 tablespoon double cream
1 tablespoon Hellmann's mayo
Pinch of paprika

CHICORY AND EGG SALAD

Remove outer leaves of chicory and finely slice
Add 2 hard-boiled eggs
Add a sprinkle of sultanas or raisins
Liquidize 2 oz fresh cream and basil and pour over the salad

DESERTS

BERRY SORBET

Liquidise and berries with spring water and freeze

CHOCOLATE DESERT

Melt one square of Green and Black's organic dark chocolate
Stir in 3 fluid ounces of double cream

CHOCOLATE STRAWBERRIES

Melt white chocolate
Dip strawberries half way and set onto a cold saucer
Allow to set
Arrange on a bed of mint and double cream

CHOCOLATE NUT NIBBLES

Lightly grease a plate with butter
Melt one slab of dark chocolate
Pour and spread over the plate (you can use grease proof paper if you wish)
Leave to set
Crush unsalted cashew nuts and sprinkle over
Melt one slab of white chocolate and then pour over
Place in fridge and leave to set, then store in airtight container

DRINKS

BANANA SMOOTHIE

Liquidise ¼ pt. Milk, 1 tablespoon double cream and one banana (other fruit can be used, not citrus)

MANGO AND BANANA SMOOTHIE

1 Banana
1 mango
¼ pt. Of organic apple juice
Liquidize

HOT CHOCOLATE

Boil one mug of milk
Stir in one square of Greer and Black's chocolate until dissolved
Add cream if required

BONE TEA

1 tsp. of comfrey and one of dried mint
Pour over boiling water and leave for 5 minutes, strain
(For healthy bones)

GINGER AND MINT OR BASIL TEA

Slice ½ inch of fresh ginger
Add ½ - 1 tspoon of mint or basil
Cover with boiling water; leave for 5 minutes then drink slowly

MISCELLANIOUS

JUST JAM

Place any berries into a pan and cover with water
Boil until the water has dissolved
Add lemon juice, store in fridge

CREAMED YAM

Grate yam using a large sized grater
Lightly fry in butter
Add double cream and salt/pepper to taste

NOTES

1. _Always soak vegetables in sea salt and water for at least 10 minutes to kill any parasites_
2.   Always rinse any items used for cooking before use to remove any airborne eggs and washing up liquid residue
3.   Always use foods that you are not allergic/intolerant to
4.   Remove all scarred and damaged areas of fruit, vegetables/food
5.   Use boiled spring water for cooking
6.   Butter is always better than spreads
7.   Most foods are available at the supermarket and farmers markets
8.   VIP do not cook at high temperatures, it makes oils toxic and damages the structure and enzymes of food
9.   Do not EVER microwave as it kills 60%+ of enzymes
10. The amounts in the menus above are for one person per serving.
11. Use Pyrex where possible
12. If you have no Pyrex saucepans, then cast iron is the next best. Do NOT use aluminium – ever or foil

SHOPPING LIST

1. Liquidizer
2. Pyrex dish and saucepans
3. Steamer
4. Non aluminium pans and cookware

FOODS TO AVOID

The Thyroid Diet gives specific details of these but in general they are:

1. all starchy foods
2. carbohydrates
3. sugars
4. fermented items
5. cheese except mozzarella
6. yeast and yeast products including brewer's yeast
7. nightshade family, potatoes, peppers etc.
8. cruciferous family – cabbage, cauliflower etc
9. fizzy drinks and cordial (make your own with a juicer)
10. tap water

Soya will also inhibit thyroid function so pleased avoid.

Other items that also affect thyroid function are: chemicals, body products, and hair dye.

SUMMARY for the best success

A SIMPLE TEST is to take your temperature before rising, if it is a degree below or more then you may be hypothyroid. Shake a glass thermometer down the night before. Upon waking place it under your armpit for ten minutes before rising, (it does take that long), if it is under 97.8F/37C you may be hypothyroid, however this may be an indication that you could also/or be hypo adrenal. Your pottering around pulse should be around 80 beats per minute; a lowered pulse rate may also be a sign of hypothyroidism. The resting pulse varies. If you are on Thyroxine/Synthroid and your resting pulse goes over 90 beats per minute you may be toxic so reduce dose by half a tablet for 4 days, if your pulse is still over 90 reduce again. Keep a diary of these and your symptoms. It also helps to keep a note of what you eat and keep a weekly activities diary.

DIET AND HORMONES
Diet plays a large part in the illness. Hypothyroids are unable to digest wheat and other grains effectively. There is often growth hormone and cortisol reduction. The wheat protein interferes with the thyroid protein. Wheat contains gluten one of the glue foods, which can cause malabsorption of nutrients. Always be food allergy and intolerance tested. Certain foods suit different blood groups. Eating incorrect foods can cause adrenal exhaustion.

SUPPLEMENTS
Most supplements are just too strong for the body, they can be toxic, and nothing compares with a good diet. KISS - keep it simple, straightforward. The golden rule is to get nutrition from food first, and buy it raw then make and cook it your self. If it is factory or industrial made it is best to avoid it. Supplements that help are: CoQ10 x 30mgs, Chromium x 200 daily, 1,000 vitamin C, Vitamin B5, and iron every second or third day.

OTHER HORMONES
These are vital for thyroid metabolism. No amount of thyroid in the blood will catalyse it into the cells without cortisol, progesterone, testosterone, pregnenolone, DHEA, and oestrogen's. You need them all to be balanced to make the metabolic system work properly. It is best to have a total hormone test.

LIST OF SIGNS AND SYMPTOMS

Underline or highlight which of these applies to you. Please remember SOME may be low adrenal function.

Physical: Exhaustion, falling asleep - wanting to go to sleep all the time, weight gain. Puffiness of: eyes, face, hands, feet, ankles. Pain in: head, migraines, lower back pain, neck pain, muscle pain, and joints aching. Cramps, pins and needles Skin: dry, flaky, course patches, sallow in colour, pallor: flushed/ normal, palms and hands red and burning, itchy hands and feet and skin generally Nails: brittle, flake off, soft   slow growing, thick toenails. Deafness, over sensitive hearing, noises in ears. Whistling in ears, aversion to loud noise. Numbness in: toes, fingers, arms, legs, back, head, (top and back) Visual disturbances: blurring, poor focusing, dry eyes, gritty eyes, sore eyes, itchy eyes, heavy (hooded) eyelids, yellow bumps on eyes. Digestive problems: Loss of appetite, food sensitivity, food allergies, wheat intolerance, problems with carbohydrate metabolism, alcohol intolerance, constipation diarrhoea, poor food absorption, pain in liver area, gassy tummy, lots of wind. Hair: loss, thinness, loss of outer third of eyebrows, lank, greasy, flat to head (no body), loss of under arm hair and pubic hair, no shine - dull falling out. Menstrual disorders: heavy periods, painful periods, loss of periods, irregular periods infertility light scant periods loss of sex drive. Slow movements, unable to walk far, low energy, slow speech. Blood pressure: high or low or normal. Dizziness, fainting feeling, palpitations, light sensitive, sun sensitive, balance problems. Intolerance of heat and cold, prone to overheating and hot flushes (flashes), feet cold, unable to get warm even with jumpers on. Insomnia. Nightmares, unable to sleep deeply and wake refreshed, (this can be liver). Snoring and sleep apnoea.

Mental: Panic attacks, poor memory especially short term, concentration poor, word confusion noises and voices in the head, hallucinations, claustrophobia, phobias, fearfulness, don't want to go out. Emotions: cry easily mood swings unable to be rational, angry, think everyone's against you. Depressed, nervous, suspicion of others motives, lack of confidence, wanting to be alone.

AFFILIATED DISEASES
Diabetes; depression, heart problems, high cholesterol, high blood pressure, problems with joints, teeth, and bones. Aching and wasting muscles. Eye disease. Hysterectomy, infertility, digestive, and colon cancer, other cancers, insanity, Alzheimer's disease; dementia. Circulation problems. Liver cancer. Chronic Fatigue Syndrome. SAD Lupus.

Hypo-adrenalism (low adrenals)

There are some general guidelines for some of the symptoms you may have. These are the runs, often late afternoon/evening this may be low adrenals. Heavy periods are often low adrenals. Light/non-existent periods may be thyroid. Constipation may also be thyroid. Headaches can be both. Back pain can be both, however if it is in the kidney region it may be adrenals, low thyroid may cause neck pain. Pain at the base of the spine is usually low thyroid. Thirst can be thyroid/adrenals. Diabetes can be thyroid/adrenals. Poor sleeping patterns can be both thyroid and adrenals. Exhaustion can be low adrenals caused by a virus, foods or parasites, or high chemicals from body products.

OTHER THINGS THAT MAKE THE THYROID SICK

Diet is 50% the cause of low thyroid function. If a person does not eat the right food, on a regular basis this can cause the person to become extremely ill. Food is medicine. The cabbage family contains chemicals called pro-goitrins which means – causes goitres i.e. makes the thyroid swell and reduces function. Starvation and excess of carbohydrates also affect thyroid function. Fats are needed – all cells contain them, hormones are made from them. Proteins are needed for normal cell production. The thyroid cell is made from 95% protein. Your hair is also 95% protein. Vegetarianism is one of the quickest routes to hypothyroidism. See The Atkins and South Beach Diets, which have sold millions of copies. You should also eat for your right blood group. The body has two responses to food it either [a] makes enzymes to break it down or [b] makes histamine for an allergic/intolerant reaction. Most people with thyroid problems have their illness based in foods and parasites/moulds/bacteria. The thyroid regulates parasites and the digestive system.

Another aspect of thyroid problems is that we are generally much too toxic. This toxicity comes from moulds, fungus, bacteria, parasites, food additives, and body products. One of the functions of the thyroid is to remove toxins from our bodies via our lymph glands, through breath, sweat, kidneys, and bowels. If you have low thyroid then this process is also reduced. Problems in these areas can be an indicator of low thyroid/low adrenals. Medicines can remain in our bodies unchanged. Deodorant and other body products really make us more toxic than we know. The aluminium in deodorant affects the thyroid. If it goes <u>onto</u> us then it goes **into** us.

Hair dye is one of the MOST toxic things to the thyroid; via the lymph it drains directly down into it. So if you die your hair and are wondering why you cannot lose weight, here is the answer. Take care with Aspirin and Warfarin, (this stops the binding of the protein and thyroid), and other over the counter medicines. The EEC is currently drawing up legislation for these products. Household and garden pesticides are near the top of the list. You can get natural hair dye. Chemicals interfere with our own natural hormone function and can cause RNA reversal in cellular reproduction. Many people have aspartame and conditioner toxicity of the pituitary gland; this in turn reduces TSH and other hormone functions.

It is important to find out what is causing the person to be ill by non-intrusive stress testing; whatever is stressed will show up clearly. Poor food types for that person will also show. Top of the stress list are foods, parasites and teeth in any order. You may have a parasite living in your thyroid, or have heavy metals lodged there, such as mercury from fillings or fluoride from toothpaste and tap water. Viruses can also live in the thyroid. A low calcium diet can be the cause. Root canals sitting on the thyroid or adrenal meridian pathways may be another reason.

Many people tested show high levels of parasites in their gut, (we all have them). These eventually get out of control. They leak through the intestine wall and get into the blood stream. Each cancer cell has a parasite living in it. Animals living in your home are a quick way to get these creatures. You should detox your animals in their food daily. (See Hulda Clark website for details). Grain mould is another food additive you really do not want to have as each time you eat grains, carbohydrates, yeast and sugar it multiplies, along with candida. Tuna parasites, turkey and beef bacteria, and parasites are the most common. The rate that aspergillus (airborne mould), is growing is showing concern in alternative health circles. We can catch this from inhaling in any location. You really do not know what is going on in your body. (For more details on toxins check out Dr. Hulda Clark's website). Do a detox twice or three times a year. This four-day detox needs to be repeated two weeks later to get rid of the eggs. Remember the thyroid controls these and the digestive system. Zapping is very successful in conjunction with the herbal detox. We all have parasites, viruses, bacteria (good and bad), and moulds living in us. Candida is also usually out of control, causing gassy tummy, bloating and frequent toilet visits.

CHEMICALS
Over 100,000 chemicals are introduced into our environment each year. They are used for many things such as in our food, to scent out rooms, body products, cleaning products etc. These chemicals interfere with our body's own production and utilisation of hormones. High chemicals users are more likely to get ill than those who use natural products. If you wouldn't drink it then don't use it. Exceptions are essential oils 100% pure – on the good side, cordial and fizzy drinks on the bad side. The only cleaning products you need are vodka, natural lemon juice, vegetable oil, salt, and bicarbonate of soda. Remember if you put it onto your skin it goes into your bloodstream. Tea tree oil is an excellent deodorant. If you wash your hair in Dove sensitive soap it becomes wonderful after a couple of weeks. Fairy non-bio, using half the recommended amount is the best washing system for clothes. Do not use conditioner, like aspartame it poisons the pituitary. These chemicals are not tested in any combination or under warm and heat conditions. Sweat doesn't smell but the bacteria that lives on it does.

Any doctor may supply natural thyroid on a private prescription. (NOTE Thyroxine is NOT natural). Natural food state thyroid is **not** made in the UK any more since 1986, and is import only – it is not in the NIMS. Take care, as it may be toxic to you - remember low doses can make things worse, and the charge should realistically be no more than £25 for 90. Most people respond to bovine better. Naturally if you have a pork allergy you may not test well for porcine thyroid, this includes Armour (porcine), which does not test as well as others. Remember low doses can make you feel worse. The usual daily dose for regular food state thyroid is 5 - 6 tablets per day. For extra strong it is 3 – 3.5 depending on your weight. Thyroid needs adrenal hormones to metabolise correctly. Bovine thyroid is freeze-dried meat from free range US/NZ cows and contains all the thyroid hormones. Each tablet of bovine is the equivalent of 25mcgs of Thyroxine. Each tablet of extra strong bovine is equivalent to 40mcgs of Synthroid or Thyroxine. Warning: this product cannot cure you but it may help with some of your signs and symptoms.

Also recommended is computerised health screening. Using hair sample analysis and DNA it is possible to check your thyroid and other hormones. It is painless, none intrusive and easy to do. Do you have food or other allergies or intolerances? (They are not the same). What parts of you are most stressed? Do your teeth cause the problem? Dead teeth in the mouth and root canal fillings can cause hypothyroidism, if they sit on that meridian. Remember the word disease comes from the body not being at ease.

Pets can also suffer from this illness and require T4 or natural thyroid supplementation.

For more information please contact: The Thyroid Support Group

Printed in Great Britain
by Amazon

23813331R00046